# How to Prevent and Reverse Heart Disease

The Step by Step Heart Healthy Easy
Recipe Cookbook for Heart Disease

ISAAC HENDRICKS

# Table of Contents

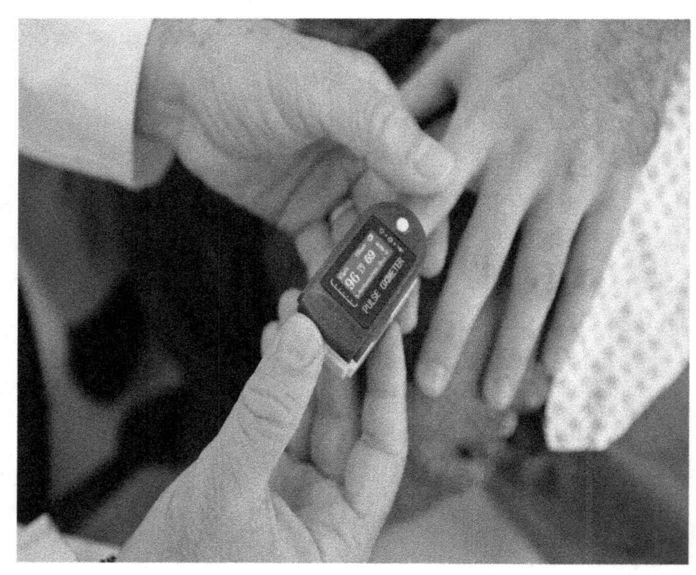

# INTRODUCTION

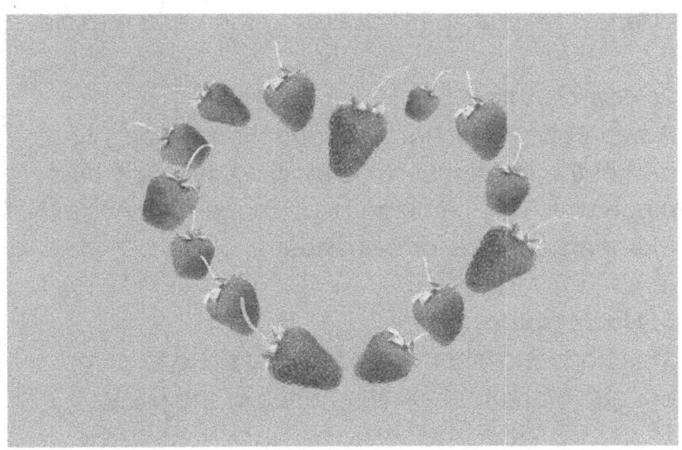

## Explanation of heart disease

Heart disease is a term that encompasses many different medical conditions that affect the heart. These conditions interfere with the normal functioning of the heart and its ability to pump blood throughout the body, resulting in various symptoms, which can lead to serious health complications and even death.

There are several different types of heart diseases, including:

**1. Coronary artery disease (CAD):**
This is the most common type of heart disease and occurs when plaque builds up in the coronary arteries, restricting blood flow to the heart muscle.

**2. Heart attack:**
A heart attack occurs when the blood supply to a part of the heart muscle is blocked, typically by a blood clot. This can lead to permanent damage to the heart muscles or even death.

**3. Heart failure:**
This happens when the heart is unable to pump enough blood to meet the needs of the body.

**4. Arrhythmia:**
This is an irregular heartbeat that can lead to dizziness, shortness of breath, and in some cases, fainting or sudden cardiac arrest.

**5. Valvular heart disease:**
This occurs when the heart valves become damaged or diseased, preventing them from opening and closing properly.

Heart disease causes differ based on the type of heart disease. However, some common risk factors include:

1. High blood pressure
2. High cholesterol
3. Obesity

4. Smoking
5. Diabetes
6. Physical inactivity
7. Family history of heart disease

Preventing heart disease involves reducing the risk factors associated with it. This includes:

1. Maintaining a healthy weight
2. Eating a balanced diet
3. Being physically active
4. Quitting smoking
5. Managing high blood pressure and cholesterol
6. Managing diabetes

Treatment of heart disease can include medication, lifestyle changes, and medical procedures such as angioplasty, stenting, or bypass surgery. Heart transplant surgery may be required in some circumstances.

In conclusion, heart disease is a serious condition that requires careful management and prevention. Knowing the types, causes, and risk factors of heart disease can help people take the necessary steps towards achieving a healthy heart and avoiding complications.

# Importance of prevention and reversal

Heart disease is one of the leading causes of death worldwide, affecting millions of individuals and their families. Prevention and reversal of heart disease is of utmost importance, as it can help reduce the number of deaths and improve overall health outcomes.

Prevention of heart disease involves adopting lifestyle changes that can reduce the risk factors associated with heart disease. These include regular exercise, a healthy diet, no smoking, limited alcohol consumption, and maintaining a healthy weight. Adopting these habits can help lower blood pressure, reduce cholesterol levels, and lower the risk of developing diabetes, all of which are significant risk factors for heart disease.

Reversal of heart disease can be achieved through medical and lifestyle interventions, depending on the severity of the condition. Medical interventions such as medications and surgical procedures can help improve heart function, reduce blockages in arteries, and prevent complications such as heart attacks and strokes. Lifestyle interventions such as regular exercise and a healthy diet can also help reverse heart disease by reducing risk factors and improving heart function.

Prevention and reversal of heart disease is of enormous importance as it can improve quality of life, increase life expectancy and reduce healthcare costs. By adopting healthy habits and seeking early medical attention, individuals can significantly reduce the risk of developing heart disease or prevent the progression of the condition if already diagnosed.

In conclusion, prevention and reversal of heart disease is paramount to reducing the burden of heart disease in society and improving overall health outcomes. It is crucial that individuals take proactive steps to adopt healthy lifestyles, seek early medical attention, and adhere to prescribed treatment plans to prevent and reverse heart disease.

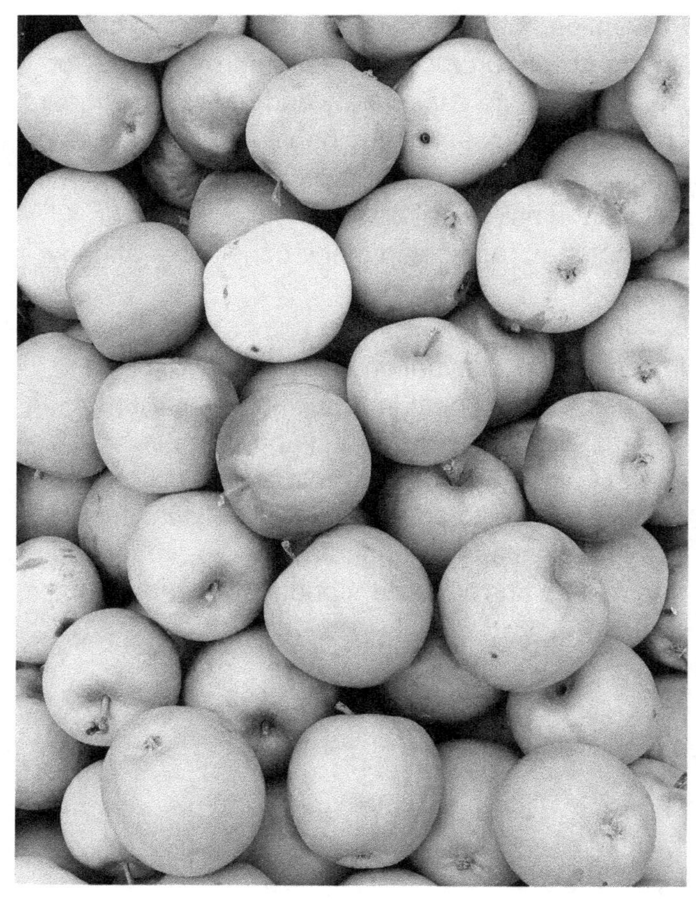

# CHAPTER ONE

## Factors Leading to Heart Disease

### Genetic predisposition

Genetic predisposition is a significant factor leading to heart disease. Heart disease, also known as cardiovascular disease, includes conditions that affect the heart and blood vessels, such as coronary artery disease, heart failure, and arrhythmias. Although lifestyle choices such as diet, physical activity, and smoking contribute to the development of heart disease, genetics play a vital role as well.

Inherited mutations or variations in genes can influence an individual's susceptibility to heart disease. For example, mutations in the LRP6, MYH6, and MYH7 genes increase the risk of developing coronary artery disease. Similarly, mutations in the PCSK9 and LPL genes can lead to high levels of LDL (bad) cholesterol, which is a significant risk factor for heart disease.

Another genetic factor that contributes to heart disease is familial hypercholesterolemia (FH), an inherited condition that causes extremely high levels of LDL cholesterol in the blood. FH increases the risk of developing coronary artery disease at a younger age, and individuals with this condition are more likely to have a heart attack or stroke.

Moreover, genetic factors can interact with environmental factors and lifestyle choices to further increase the risk of heart disease. For example, an individual with a genetic predisposition to heart disease who smokes or has an unhealthy diet is at a higher risk of developing the condition.

In conclusion, genetic predisposition is a crucial factor leading to heart disease. Identifying genetic mutations and variants that increase the risk of heart disease can help healthcare professionals develop targeted prevention and treatment strategies. Additionally, individuals with a family history of heart disease should be aware of their increased risk and take measures to minimise their risk factors.

## Lifestyle Choices

Heart disease is a serious condition that affects millions of people around the world and is a leading cause of death in many countries. It is caused by various factors, including lifestyle choices that can increase the risk of developing heart disease over time. Here are some lifestyle choices that can increase the risk of heart disease.

**1. Poor Diet:**
A diet high in saturated and trans fats, salt, and cholesterol and low in fruits, vegetables, and fibre can lead to the development of heart disease over time. Consuming excessive amounts of sugar and artificial sweeteners can also increase the risk of developing heart disease. Processed and fast foods are also high in unhealthy fats and salt which increase the risk.

**2. Lack of Physical Activity:**
A sedentary lifestyle where individuals spend most of their day sitting, lying down, or participating in low-intensity activities can increase the risk of heart disease over time. Regular exercise is essential for maintaining good heart health as it keeps the muscles of the heart healthy and helps to maintain a healthy weight.

**3. Smoking:**
Smoking cigarettes is one of the most significant lifestyle choices leading to heart disease. The chemicals in cigarettes damage the lining of the arteries, which can cause plaque buildup and blood clots, leading to heart attacks.

**4. Excessive Alcohol Consumption:** Drinking too much alcohol can lead to high blood pressure, which increases the risk of developing heart disease. Heavy drinking can also lead to atrial fibrillation and a weakened heart muscle, increasing the risk of heart failure.

**5. Stress:**
Chronic stress triggers the production of stress hormones that can lead to high blood pressure and increased heart rate, which, over time, can damage the heart muscle and increase the risk of heart disease.

In conclusion, adopting a healthy lifestyle and making changes to diet and activity level can reduce the risk of heart disease. It is essential to maintain a balanced and nutritious diet, engage in regular physical activity, stop smoking, limit alcohol consumption and manage stress levels for a healthy heart.

## Medical conditions

Heart disease refers to a variety of heart-related illnesses, including coronary artery disease, heart failure, and arrhythmias. Medical conditions are major factors that can lead to heart disease. Some of these conditions are:

**1. High blood pressure:**
High blood pressure or hypertension increases the workload on the heart and can damage the blood vessels leading to the heart. This can cause atherosclerosis, a condition where the arteries become narrow and limit blood flow to the heart.

**2. High cholesterol:**

High levels of low-density lipoprotein (LDL) cholesterol can build up on the walls of arteries, forming plaque. This can also lead to atherosclerosis and increase the risk of heart disease.

### 3. Diabetes:
Diabetes can damage blood vessels and nerves, leading to complications such as atherosclerosis and peripheral artery disease. It can also increase the risk of hypertension and excessive cholesterol.

### 4. Obesity:
Obesity increases the risk of high blood pressure, high cholesterol, and diabetes, all of which can increase the risk of heart disease.

### 5. Sleep apnea:
Sleep apnea is a condition where breathing is interrupted during sleep, leading to low oxygen levels and increased blood pressure. This can increase the risk of heart disease, especially in those with existing high blood pressure or diabetes.

### 6. Rheumatoid arthritis:
Rheumatoid arthritis is an autoimmune disorder that can cause inflammation and damage to blood vessels and the heart. This can raise the likelihood of developing heart disease.

### 7. Kidney disease:

Chronic kidney disease can lead to high blood pressure and damage to blood vessels, increasing the risk of heart disease.

**8. Congenital heart defects:**
Some individuals are born with heart defects that can lead to complications later in life, such as an increased risk of heart disease.

In conclusion, managing medical conditions can significantly reduce the risk of developing heart disease. It's important to seek medical attention when symptoms arise, and to follow a healthy lifestyle with regular exercise, a healthy diet and a cessation of smoking for people who smoke.

# CHAPTER TWO

## How to Prevent Heart Disease

### Healthy diet

Cardiovascular diseases such as heart attack, stroke, and coronary artery disease are some of the leading causes of death worldwide. However, research has shown that a healthy diet can significantly reduce your risk of developing heart disease and even help you manage existing heart health conditions. Here is a guide on healthy diets to control heart disease:

### 1. Emphasise on whole foods

Fruits, vegetables, whole grains, nuts, legumes, and lean proteins are rich in nutrients that promote heart health. These foods are also low in saturated fats, trans fats, and cholesterol that increase the risk of heart disease. Aim for a wide variety of colourful fresh fruits and vegetables to get a range of nutrients.

### 2. Minimise Salt

Eating too much salt can cause high blood pressure- a major risk factor for heart disease. Processed foods, as well as deep-fried foods, often have high levels of sodium, so try to limit your intake of these foods. Instead, use natural herbs, spices, and citrus juices to add flavour to your meals.

## 3. Reduce unhealthy fats

Trans fats, saturated fats, and dietary cholesterol raise blood cholesterol levels, which increases the risk for heart disease. Minimise your intake of red meat, processed meats, cheese, fried foods, butter, and margarine.

## 4. Choose healthy fats

Monounsaturated fats and polyunsaturated fats are considered "healthy fats" that are good for your heart health. You can find these fats in foods such as nuts, seeds, avocados, fatty fish, and vegetable oils like olive oil. Including them in your diet helps in reducing the chances of heart attacks and strokes.

## 5. Watch portion sizes

Eating too much of anything, even healthy food, can lead to weight gain and other health problems. Stick to recommended portion sizes and focus on eating balanced meals with plenty of whole foods and lean protein.

In conclusion, choosing healthy food choices and a diet rich in whole foods, fruits, vegetables, nuts, lean protein, healthy fats, and whole grains can help control heart disease. You should not put all your eggs in one basket, other lifestyle factors like maintaining an active life, controlling stress, and getting adequate sleep are also vital in controlling heart disease.

## Regular exercise

Regular exercise has been identified as one of the most critical factors in controlling heart disease. According to medical experts, heart disease is one of the leading causes of death globally, with lifestyle choices, including physical inactivity, being a significant risk factor.

Physical activity and exercises have been found to positively impact and help in reducing the risk of heart-related complications drastically. Regular workouts and physical activities are known to improve blood circulation, reduce blood pressure, and improve metabolism. Additionally, engaging in regular exercise also helps in reducing body weight, which, in turn, reduces the risk associated with obesity, such as stroke and heart diseases.

Experts recommend that adults engage in at least 150 minutes of moderate aerobic exercise per week, preferably in 30-minute sessions at least five times per week. For individuals with pre-existing heart-related conditions, it is essential to consult with a healthcare professional before commencing a physical exercise regimen.

In conclusion, regular exercise is a vital component in preventing and reducing the risk of heart disease. Engaging in regular physical activities such as walking, cycling, swimming, weight training, and other forms of aerobic exercise can significantly lower the likelihood of developing heart diseases. Therefore, it is essential to incorporate regular physical exercise in our daily routine for overall heart health and wellness.

## Eliminating bad habits

Eliminating bad habits is an essential part of controlling heart disease. The following are some tips that may help in getting rid of harmful habits to keep the heart healthy:

1. Quit smoking- Smoking is a major risk factor for heart disease. It is essential to quit smoking and stay away from secondhand smoke as well.

2. Engage in regular exercise- sedentary lifestyle is another risk factor for heart disease. Engaging in regular physical activity helps to keep the heart healthy and also helps to control other risk factors like high blood pressure and high cholesterol levels.

3. Avoid unhealthy food choices- consuming unhealthy foods like processed foods, high sodium foods, and high-fat foods can increase the risk of heart disease. It is essential to make healthy food choices like eating fresh fruits, vegetables, whole grains, lean meats, and healthy fats.

4. Manage stress- chronic stress can lead to high blood pressure, which is a significant risk factor for heart disease. Finding ways to manage stress like meditation, yoga, or breathing exercises can be helpful.

5. Limit alcohol consumption- excessive alcohol consumption can lead to high blood pressure and other heart-related issues. It is essential to limit alcohol intake to a moderate level.

In conclusion, eliminating bad habits is crucial in controlling heart disease. Adopting healthy habits like quitting smoking, engaging in regular exercise, making healthy food choices, managing stress, and limiting alcohol intake can be effective in keeping the heart healthy.

## Managing stress

Stress plays a crucial role in the development and progression of heart disease. Therefore, managing stress is critical for controlling heart disease. Here are some ways to manage stress to control heart disease:

**1. Exercise on a regular basis:** Exercise is one of the most effective stress-reduction methods. Exercise releases endorphins, which help to reduce stress hormones in the body. Regular exercise also helps to strengthen the heart and improve overall cardiovascular health.

**2. Practice relaxation techniques:** There are many relaxation techniques that you can practice to reduce stress, such as deep breathing, meditation, yoga, and Tai Chi. These techniques help to calm the mind and body and reduce the physical symptoms of stress.

**3. Maintain a healthy diet:** A healthy diet can help to reduce stress levels and improve cardiovascular health. Consume plenty of fruits and vegetables, whole grains, lean protein, and healthy fats.

**4. Get enough sleep:** Lack of sleep can lead to increased stress levels and worsen heart disease symptoms. Aim for seven to eight hours of sleep every night to feel well-rested and refreshed.

**5. Seek support:** Talking to a friend, family member, or therapist can help to alleviate stress and provide emotional support. Joining a support group for individuals with heart disease can also be helpful.

In conclusion, managing stress is critical for controlling heart disease. Implementing these stress management strategies can help to reduce stress levels and improve overall cardiovascular health.

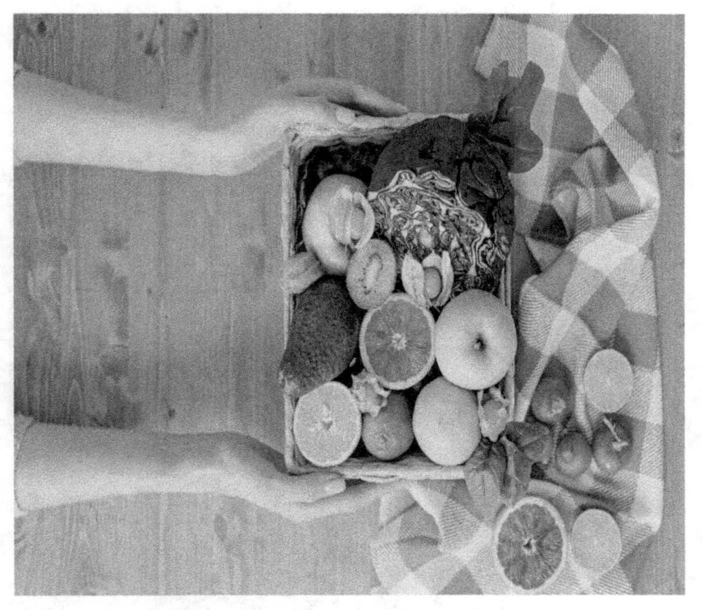

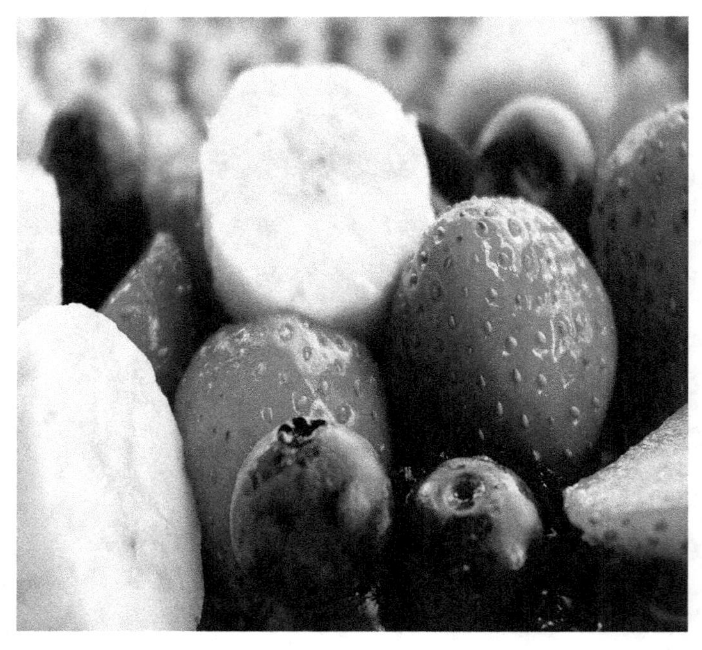

# CHAPTER THREE

## How to Reverse Heart Disease

### Medical treatments

A combination of disorders affecting the heart and blood arteries is referred to as heart disease, often known as cardiovascular disease. These conditions can lead to various health complications, such as heart attack, stroke, heart failure, and kidney damage. However, there are several medical treatments that can help to reverse or manage heart disease.

### 1. Medications:

A range of medications can be used to manage heart disease, including blood thinners, cholesterol-lowering drugs, beta-blockers, and ACE inhibitors. These medications work to help reduce the risk of heart attack and stroke and can help to control high blood pressure and other symptoms.

### 2. Lifestyle changes:

Adopting a healthy lifestyle is crucial for managing heart disease. This includes eating a balanced and healthy diet that is low in saturated fat, salt, and sugar. Additionally, regular exercise can help to lower blood pressure, reduce cholesterol levels, and improve heart function.

### 3. Cardiac rehabilitation:

Cardiac rehabilitation is a program that consists of supervised exercise, education, counselling, and support sessions designed to help people recover from heart disease. This program can help to improve cardiovascular health and prevent future heart disease complications.

### 4. Medical procedures:

In some cases, medical procedures may be necessary to help reverse or manage heart disease. These procedures include angioplasty, heart valve repair or replacement, and coronary artery bypass surgery. These procedures can help to improve blood flow to the heart and improve its function.

In conclusion, there are several medical treatments available to reverse or manage heart disease. These treatments include medications, lifestyle changes, cardiac rehabilitation, and medical procedures. However, it is important to work with a healthcare professional to determine the best treatment plan for your individual needs and circumstances.

## Lifestyle changes

Heart disease is a chronic condition caused by a buildup of plaque in the arteries, resulting in reduced blood flow to the heart. Adopting a healthy lifestyle can help reverse heart disease and prevent further damage.

### 1. Quit smoking:
Smoking is a major risk factor for heart disease. Quitting smoking lowers the risk immediately and promotes better health.

### 2. Exercise regularly:
Exercise helps improve blood circulation, reduces stress, and strengthens the heart muscle. Five days a week, thirty minutes of moderate-intensity exercise is recommended.

### 3. Eat a heart-healthy diet:
A diet rich in fruits, vegetables, whole grains, lean proteins, and low-fat dairy products can help to improve heart health.

### 4. Manage stress:
Stress can raise blood pressure and trigger inflammation, leading to heart disease. Relaxation techniques such as yoga, meditation, deep breathing, and regular exercise can help to manage stress.

### 5. Maintain a healthy weight:
Being overweight or obese increases the risk of developing heart disease. Weight loss with a nutritious diet and regular exercise can help lower the risk.

**6. Get enough sleep:**
Sleep plays an important role in overall health and well-being. Getting enough sleep (7-9 hours per night) can help reduce the risk of heart disease.

**7. Manage underlying health conditions:**
High blood pressure, high cholesterol, and diabetes are all risk factors for heart disease. Managing these conditions through diet, exercise, and medication can help improve heart health.

By adopting a healthier lifestyle, you can help to reverse heart disease or prevent it from developing. It's never too late to make positive lifestyle changes that benefit your heart and overall health.

## Dietary modifications

While there are many risk factors that contribute to the development of heart disease, such as genetic factors, age, and smoking, dietary factors also play an important role. By making dietary modifications, individuals can effectively manage, and in some cases reverse, heart disease.

Here are some dietary modifications that can help reverse heart disease:

### 1. Eat a diet rich in plant-based foods:

Consuming a diet that is high in fruits, vegetables, legumes, and whole grains can help improve heart health by reducing cholesterol levels and inflammation in the body. Plant-based diets have also been shown to lower blood pressure, improve insulin sensitivity, and reduce the risk of heart disease.

## 2. Reduce saturated fat intake:

Saturated fats found in red meat, dairy products, and certain oils can increase cholesterol levels and contribute to the development of heart disease. Replace saturated fats with unsaturated fats such as olive oil, avocados, nuts, seeds, and fatty fish like salmon, which can help lower cholesterol levels and improve heart health.

## 3. Limit sodium intake:

High sodium intake can lead to high blood pressure, which is a major risk factor for heart disease. Limiting sodium intake to less than 2,300 milligrams per day (or 1,500 milligrams per day for those with high blood pressure) and avoiding processed and fast foods that are high in sodium can help improve heart health.

## 4. Increase omega-3 fatty acid intake:

Omega-3 fatty acids found in fatty fish, flaxseeds, and walnuts have been shown to reduce inflammation, lower triglyceride levels, and improve heart health. Incorporate sources of omega-3 fatty acids into your diet to help prevent or reverse heart disease.

Processed foods that are high in sugar, salt, and unhealthy fats can contribute to the development of heart disease. Instead, choose whole, unprocessed foods such as fresh fruits, vegetables, and whole grains, which can help improve heart health.

In conclusion, making dietary modifications can significantly improve heart health and even reverse heart disease. Incorporating a plant-based diet, reducing saturated fat and sodium intake, increasing omega-3 fatty acid intake, and avoiding processed and sugary foods can help individuals manage and prevent heart disease. Consult a healthcare provider for personalised dietary recommendations and guidance.

## Supplemental therapies

Supplemental therapies can be used in conjunction with conventional treatments to reverse or slow down the progression of heart disease. These therapies are generally safe and can have positive effects on overall health. Here are some of the most effective supplemental therapies to reverse heart disease:

**1. Fish Oil Supplements:**
Omega-3 fatty acids found in fish oil have been shown to improve lipid profiles, reduce inflammation, and lower the risk of heart disease.

**2. Coenzyme Q10 Supplements:**
This enzyme is vital for energy production in the
body and also acts as an antioxidant. CoQ10
supplementation has been shown to reduce the
incidence of major cardiovascular events.

**3. Magnesium Supplements:**
Magnesium is required for proper muscle and nerve
function. Supplementation with magnesium can
improve blood pressure, reduce arterial stiffness,
and improve insulin sensitivity.

**4. Exercise:**
Regular exercise is crucial in maintaining a healthy
heart. Cardiovascular exercise can improve
circulation, reduce inflammation, and improve
mood.

**5. Acupuncture:**
This ancient practice has been shown to lower
blood pressure, reduce stress levels, and improve
overall heart function.

**6. Meditation:**
Practising mindfulness meditation has been shown
to reduce stress hormone levels, lower blood
pressure, and improve overall heart health.

Supplemental therapies can be an effective way to
prevent and reverse heart disease. It is important to
consult with a healthcare professional before
starting any new supplement or exercise program.

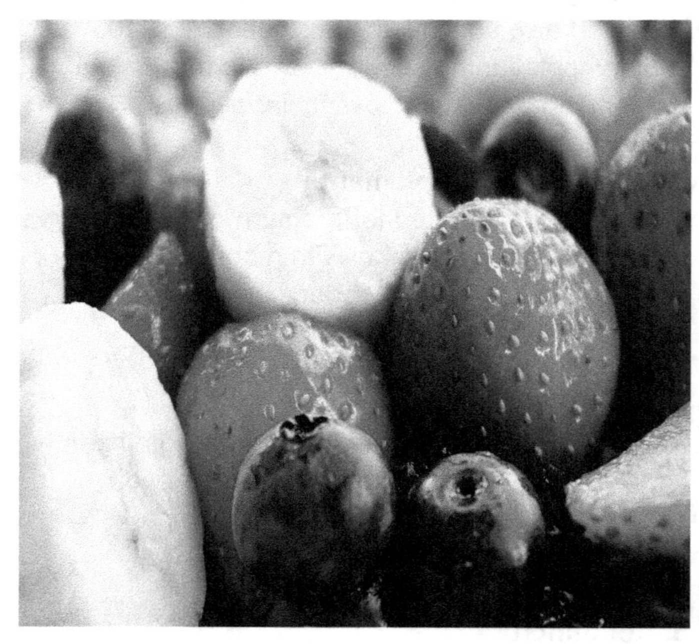

# CHAPTER FOUR

## Understanding Cholesterol and Triglycerides

### Explanation of types of cholesterol

Cholesterol is a waxy, fat-like substance that is naturally produced by our body and is vital for the formation of cell membranes and the production of hormones and other important molecules. Having too much cholesterol in the blood, on the other hand, can increase the risk of heart disease and stroke.

Low-density lipoprotein (LDL) and high-density lipoprotein (HDL) are the two main kinds of cholesterol.

### 1. LDL Cholesterol:

LDL cholesterol is often called "bad" cholesterol because it can build up in the walls of arteries, leading to the formation of plaque that can narrow arteries and increase the risk of heart disease. LDL cholesterol levels should be kept low and ideally should be less than 100 mg/dL, according to the American Heart Association.

HDL cholesterol is often referred to as "good" cholesterol because it helps remove LDL cholesterol from the arteries and carries it back to the liver, where it can be processed and eliminated from the body. Higher levels of HDL cholesterol are associated with a lower risk of heart disease, and levels above 60 mg/dL are considered to be protective.

In addition to LDL and HDL cholesterol, there is also a type of cholesterol called triglycerides, which are a type of fat found in the blood. Elevated triglyceride levels can also increase the risk of heart disease.

To reduce the risk of high cholesterol levels and heart disease, it is important to maintain healthy lifestyle habits including regular exercise, healthy diet, maintaining a healthy weight, and avoiding smoking and excessive alcohol consumption. If cholesterol levels are elevated, medication may be prescribed by a healthcare provider to help lower levels.

## Explanation of Triglycerides

Triglycerides are a type of lipid or fat that are present in our bodies and food. They are made up of three fatty acid chains connected to a glycerol backbone. Triglycerides are the main form of fat stored in our adipose tissues and are also found in our bloodstream.

Triglycerides are primarily obtained from the foods we eat, including fatty meats, whole milk, cheese, butter, oils, nuts, and seeds. Our liver can also produce triglycerides, especially after a high-carbohydrate, high-sugar meal.

The function of triglycerides is to store energy that can be used by our cells in times of need. Triglycerides can be broken down into fatty acids and glycerol by enzymes called lipases, which can then be used by cells to generate energy.

High levels of triglycerides in the bloodstream are associated with several health risks, including heart disease, stroke, and type 2 diabetes. High triglyceride levels can be caused by genetics, an unhealthy diet, sedentary lifestyle, excessive alcohol intake, and certain medical conditions like obesity, metabolic syndrome, and thyroid disorders.

To lower triglyceride levels, lifestyle modifications like weight loss, regular exercise, and a healthy diet low in saturated fat and carbohydrates are recommended. Medications like fibrates, niacin, and statins may also be prescribed in certain cases to lower triglyceride levels.

In summary, triglycerides are a type of fat that are essential for energy storage and metabolism in our bodies. However, high levels of triglycerides can be associated with health problems, and it is important to maintain a healthy lifestyle and seek medical attention if triglyceride levels are high.

# CHAPTER FIVE

## Healthy Diet for Heart Health

### Foods to include

A healthy diet is crucial for a healthy heart. The following foods are excellent sources of nutrients that promote heart health:

**1. Oily fish:**
Fatty fish, such as salmon, mackerel, and sardines, are rich in omega-3 fatty acids, which reduce inflammation and lower blood pressure and triglyceride levels.

**2. Nuts and seeds:**
Almonds, walnuts, chia seeds, and flaxseeds are high in omega-3 fatty acids, fibre, and other nutrients that support heart health.

**3. Whole grains:**
Whole grains, such as oats, barley, and quinoa, are rich in fiber, which lowers cholesterol levels and reduces the risk of heart disease.

**4. Fruits and vegetables:**
Fruits and vegetables are high in antioxidants, fibre, and other nutrients that keep the heart healthy. Berries, leafy greens, tomatoes, and citrus fruits are especially nutritious.

**5. Legumes:**
Beans, lentils, chickpeas, and peas are excellent sources of protein, fibre, and other nutrients that reduce the risk of heart disease.

**6. Avocado:**
Avocado is rich in healthy monounsaturated fats, fibre, and potassium, which lower cholesterol levels and prevent heart disease.

**7. Low-fat dairy:**
Low-fat dairy, such as yoghurt, cheese, and milk, are rich in calcium and other nutrients that promote heart health.

**8. Dark chocolate:**
Dark chocolate is rich in flavonoids, which reduce inflammation and improve heart health.

By including a variety of these heart-healthy foods in your diet, you can keep your heart healthy and reduce the risk of heart disease.

## Foods to avoid

Eating a healthy diet is crucial for maintaining good heart health. One of the best ways to promote heart health is to limit foods that are high in saturated or trans fats, cholesterol, salt, and added sugars. Here are some foods to avoid or limit for a healthier heart:

**1. Fried foods:**
Fried foods are usually high in trans fats and saturated fats, which can raise cholesterol levels and increase the risk of heart disease.

**2. Processed meats:**
Processed meats, such as deli meats, hot dogs, and sausages, are high in salt and saturated fats. They have also been linked to an increased risk of heart disease.

**3. Sugary drinks:**
Sugary drinks, such as sports drinks, energy drinks, and soda, are high in added sugars that can contribute to weight gain, insulin resistance, and high blood sugar levels.

**4. High-sugar foods:**
Foods that contain added sugars, such as desserts, pastries, and candy, should be avoided or limited. These foods can increase the risk of obesity, type 2 diabetes, and heart disease.

**5. Salt:**
High-salt foods, such as canned soups, packaged snacks, and processed foods, can increase blood pressure and put a strain on the heart.

**6. Red meat:**

Red meat, such as beef and pork, is high in saturated fats, which can increase cholesterol levels and the risk of heart disease.

**7. Dairy products:**
Some dairy products, such as cheese and butter, are high in saturated fats and should be eaten in moderation.

By avoiding these foods and opting for a diet rich in fruits, vegetables, whole grains, nuts, and lean proteins, you can promote heart health and reduce the risk of heart disease.

## Nutrient needs

Maintaining a healthy heart is key to overall health and well-being. One way to do this is by eating a well-balanced diet rich in nutrients that support heart health. The following are some essential nutrients to include in your diet:

**1. Omega-3 fatty acids:**
These are found in fatty fish such as salmon, tuna, and mackerel. Omega-3 fatty acids can help reduce inflammation, lower blood pressure, and decrease the risk of developing heart disease.

**2. Fibre:**
A diet rich in fibre can help lower cholesterol levels and reduce the risk of heart disease. Fruits,

vegetables, whole grains, and legumes are high in
fibre.

### 3. Potassium:
This mineral can help regulate blood pressure and
reduce the risk of stroke. Good sources of
potassium include bananas, oranges, leafy greens,
and white potatoes with the skin on.

### 4. Magnesium:
This mineral can help regulate heart rhythm and
reduce the risk of heart disease. Good sources of
magnesium include nuts, seeds, spinach, and black
beans.

### 5. Antioxidants:
These are found in fruits and vegetables and can
help reduce inflammation and oxidative stress,
which can contribute to heart disease. Good
sources of antioxidants include berries, tomatoes,
leafy greens, and bell peppers.

It's important to note that a well-balanced diet is key
to achieving optimal heart health. This includes
consuming a variety of nutrient-dense foods in
appropriate portions and limiting intake of
processed and high-fat foods. Consult with a
healthcare professional or registered dietitian to
develop an individualised eating plan to support
your heart health.

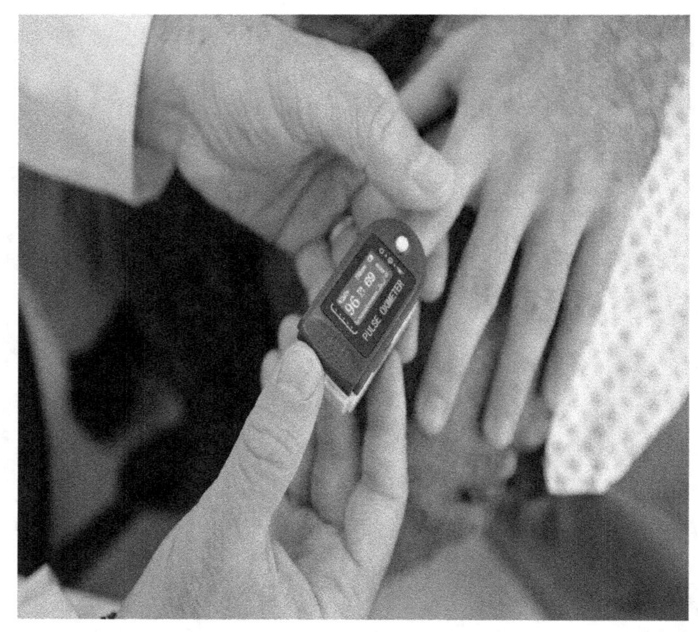


96
PULSE OXIMETER

# CHAPTER SIX

## Regular Exercise for Heart Health

### Types of exercise

Regular exercise is essential for maintaining overall heart health. There are several types of exercises that can help improve cardiovascular fitness, reduce the risk of heart disease, and strengthen the heart muscles. Here are some of the most beneficial types of exercise for heart health:

### Aerobic Exercise:

Also known as cardiovascular exercise, this type of exercise increases heart rate and improves lung function. It includes activities such as brisk walking, jogging, swimming, cycling, dancing, and aerobics. These exercises strengthen the heart muscle, lower blood pressure, and improve circulation.

### Strength Training:

Building muscle strength through resistance exercises not only improves overall body strength but also contributes to heart health. Strength training can be done using free weights, weight machines, resistance bands, or bodyweight exercises like push-ups, squats, or lunges. It helps improve overall body composition, reduces body fat, and assists in managing weight and blood sugar levels.

## High-Intensity Interval Training (HIIT):

HIIT workouts involve alternating between short bursts of intense exercise and brief periods of rest or lower-intensity activity. HIIT exercises can include sprinting, jumping jacks, burpees, or cycling at maximum intensity for a short duration. These workouts are highly effective in improving cardiovascular fitness, increasing endurance, and boosting metabolism.

## Flexibility and Stretching Exercises:

Stretching exercises like yoga and Pilates help improve flexibility, reduce muscle tension, enhance posture, and promote relaxation. While flexibility exercises are not directly linked to heart health, they indirectly contribute by improving overall fitness, preventing injuries, and enabling other forms of exercise.

## Low-Impact Exercises:

For individuals with joint problems or those who cannot perform high-impact activities, low-impact exercises provide an excellent alternative. Examples include walking, cycling, swimming, water aerobics, or using an elliptical machine. These exercises are gentle on the joints, yet still help improve cardiovascular fitness and strength.

It is important to consult a healthcare professional before starting any new exercise routine, especially for individuals with pre-existing health conditions. They can provide personalised recommendations and guidelines based on an individual's specific needs and health goals. Remember, consistency is key, and combining different types of exercise can optimise heart health and promote overall well-being.

## Frequency and intensity

Frequency and intensity play crucial roles in maintaining good heart health. Regular exercise at a moderate intensity can significantly reduce the risk of cardiovascular diseases, such as heart attack and stroke. The American Heart Association advises 150 minutes per week of moderate-intensity aerobic activity or 75 minutes per week of vigorous-intensity aerobic exercise.

Frequency refers to how often you exercise. It is important to aim for consistency and regularity in your exercise routine to derive maximum benefits for your heart. It is recommended to exercise at least three to five times a week to maintain good heart health.

Intensity refers to the level of effort you put into your exercise activity. The intensity of exercise is usually measured using maximum heart rate or perceived exertion rate. Moderate-intensity exercise, such as brisk walking, cycling, or swimming, should be enough to increase heart rate and breathing rate, but still allow you to carry on a conversation. Vigorous-intensity exercise, such as running, fast-paced cycling, or HIIT (high-intensity interval training), should raise your heart rate and breathing rate significantly and make it challenging to maintain a conversation.

In summary, the frequency and intensity of your exercise routine are important factors in maintaining good heart health. Consistency and regularity in moderate-to-high intensity aerobic exercise can reduce the risk of heart disease and improve overall heart health.

## Mind-body practices

Heart health is a critical aspect of overall fitness and wellbeing of an individual. It is essential to maintain a healthy heart to function optimally and prevent the risk of heart diseases. Mind-body practices are a set of activities that combine physical and mental exercises to promote wellness and health. These practices can help in controlling stress, physical activity, and improving cardiovascular health. Some of the popular mind-body practices for heart health are:

**1. Yoga:**
It is a low-impact physical activity that can help lower blood pressure, reduce stress, and

strengthen the heart. Yoga poses such as the plank, downward-facing dog, and warrior pose can improve the overall strength of the body and promote cardiovascular health.

**2. Tai Chi:**
It is a gentle form of martial art that involves slow and controlled movements. Tai chi can reduce stress, improve balance, and lower blood pressure, which can benefit the heart.

**3. Meditation:**
It is a relaxation technique that involves focusing on the present moment to control stress and anxiety. Meditation can reduce blood pressure, improve heart rate variability, and promote overall cardiovascular health.

**4. Breathing exercises:**
Deep breathing techniques such as diaphragmatic breathing and alternate nostril breathing can reduce stress, lower blood pressure, and improve heart function.

**5. Mindfulness practices:**
Mindfulness involves being present in the moment and paying attention to thoughts and feelings without judgement. It can reduce stress, lower blood pressure, and improve overall cardiovascular health.

In conclusion, mind-body practices can provide substantial benefits for heart health. Incorporating these practices into daily life can help manage stress, improve physical activity, and promote cardiovascular health.

# CHAPTER SEVEN

## Managing Stress for Heart Health

Meditation and mindfulness

Meditation and mindfulness have been shown to have numerous benefits for heart health. Chronic stress, anxiety, and depression have been linked to a greater risk of heart disease, and meditation could be a preventative measure for managing these mental health conditions.

Mindfulness meditation involves focusing your attention on the present moment, without judgement. By doing so, it teaches you to let go of negative thoughts and emotions that may trigger stress.

A study published in the Journal of the American College of Cardiology suggests that meditation can decrease one's blood pressure, leading to a reduced risk of heart attack or stroke. Several other studies have also shown that meditation and mindfulness can help reduce stress and anxiety levels and improve sleep quality, which can in turn lead to a healthier heart.

One particular form of meditation, called Transcendental Meditation, has been found to reduce the risk of heart attack and stroke by nearly

50% in those who practised it compared to individuals who did not meditate.

Additionally, meditation and mindfulness have been shown to promote healthier lifestyle choices like a healthy diet, regular exercise, and smoking cessation, which are all crucial for maintaining good heart health.

In conclusion, meditation and mindfulness are powerful tools that can improve heart health and reduce the risk of heart disease. Including meditation and mindfulness practices in daily life can lead to significant heart hrelaxationealth benefits.

## Yoga and other relaxation techniques

Yoga and other  techniques can be highly beneficial for heart health. In today's fast-paced lifestyle, it's common for people to suffer from stress and anxiety, which can be detrimental to overall health, including heart health. Stress and anxiety can lead to high blood pressure, increased heart rate, and other cardiovascular diseases.

Yoga, along with other relaxation techniques such as meditation and deep breathing, can help to manage stress and anxiety. Research has shown that practising yoga regularly can lower blood pressure, help regulate heartbeat, and improve circulation, all of which positively impact heart health.

Some specific yoga poses that can be beneficial for heart health include:

1. Tadasana (Mountain Pose) - helps to improve posture and circulation

2. Uttanasana (Standing Forward Bend) - can help to lower blood pressure and reduce stress

3. Trikonasana (Triangle Pose) - improves circulation and strengthens the heart and lungs

4. Bhujangasana (Cobra Pose) - can help to reduce stress and anxiety

Along with yoga, deep breathing exercises can also help to reduce stress and regulate breathing, both of which can positively impact heart health. One such exercise is called "Box Breathing," where you inhale for a count of four, hold for a count of four, exhale for a count of four, and then hold for a count of four again.

In conclusion, incorporating yoga and other relaxation techniques into daily life can help to promote heart health by reducing stress and anxiety, regulating blood pressure and heartbeat, and improving circulation. Practising these techniques regularly can lead to a healthier heart and overall well-being.

## Counselling and therapy

Counselling and therapy can play a vital role in promoting heart health. By addressing issues such as stress, anxiety, depression, and unhealthy coping behaviours, individuals can improve their emotional well-being and reduce their risk of heart disease.

One of the primary ways counselling can help is by addressing stress management. Chronic stress can lead to increased blood pressure, inflammation, and other risk factors for heart disease. Counselling can teach individuals healthy ways to manage stress, such as relaxation techniques, mindfulness, and time management skills.

Therapy can also address unhealthy coping behaviours like smoking, overeating, and excessive alcohol consumption. Counsellors can work with individuals to develop healthier coping mechanisms, such as exercise, healthy eating habits, social support, and hobbies. Making these lifestyle changes can reduce the risk of heart disease and improve overall well-being.

In addition, counselling can help individuals with existing heart conditions, such as heart attack survivors and those with heart failure, to manage their emotions and improve their quality of life. Through counselling, individuals can learn how to cope with anxiety, depression, and other emotional challenges that often come with heart disease.

Overall, counselling and therapy can be an important part of heart health management. By providing emotional support, stress management, and healthy lifestyle advice, counsellors can help individuals reduce their risk of heart disease and improve their quality of life.

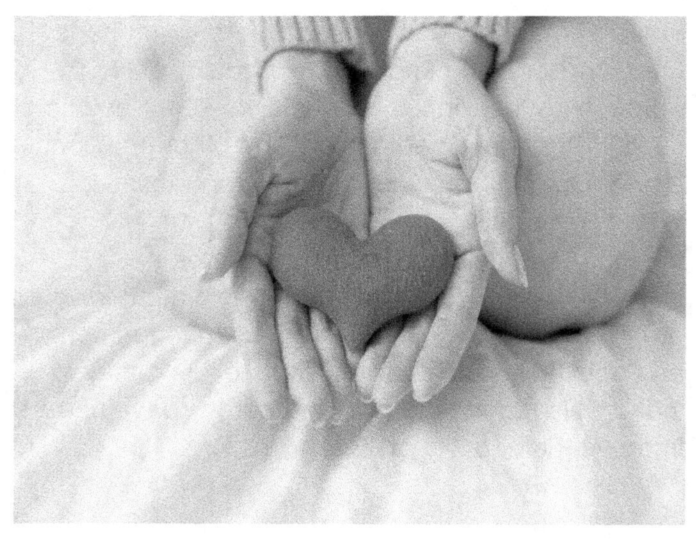

# CHAPTER EIGHT

## Supplemental Therapies for Heart Health

### Alternative therapies

Heart disease is a major concern worldwide, and various medical treatments, including drugs, surgeries, and lifestyle modifications, have been developed to address the condition. However, there is growing interest in alternative therapies, which are non-medical approaches to promoting heart health. Some of these supplemental alternative therapies for heart health are as follows:

**1. Acupuncture:** This traditional Chinese medicine technique involves inserting thin needles into specific points on the skin to improve blood flow and reduce stress, which can lower blood pressure and improve heart function.

**2. Yoga:** Yoga is a practice that combines physical postures, breathing exercises, and meditation. It has been found to reduce stress levels, which can help lower blood pressure and decrease the risk of heart disease.

**3. Meditation:** Meditation is a technique that involves training the mind to focus and calm down.

The practice has been found to reduce stress, lower blood pressure, and reduce the risk of heart disease.

**4. Chiropractic Care:** This is a complementary and alternative medicine technique that involves manipulating the spine to improve spinal alignment and nervous system function, which can promote heart health.

**5. Nutrition therapy:** A balanced, healthy diet is essential for heart health. A nutrition therapist can provide individualised advice on specific foods and supplements that affect heart function and reduce the risk of heart disease.

**6. Massage therapy:** This type of therapy involves manipulating soft tissues in the body to promote relaxation and reduce stress, which can lead to lower blood pressure and a decreased risk of heart disease.

**7. Tai Chi:** This martial art form combines slow movements with deep breathing and meditation. Tai Chi has been found to reduce stress, lower blood pressure, and improve heart function.

While alternative therapies may not replace traditional medical interventions for heart health, they can be used in combination with these treatments to promote overall wellness and improve heart function. Before beginning any alternative therapy, it is critical to consult with a healthcare provider.

## Herbal Remedies

Heart health is critical to living a healthy life. Our heart pumps blood throughout the body and provides essential nutrients and oxygen to all organs. Several herbal remedies can help promote heart health by improving blood circulation, reducing cholesterol levels, and preventing high blood pressure. In this article, we will discuss some popular herbal remedies for heart health:

**1. Hawthorn:** Hawthorn is a popular herb known for its ability to improve heart health. It helps dilate blood vessels and promotes blood circulation to the heart, reducing the risk of heart attack and stroke. Hawthorn can also lower blood pressure, reduce cholesterol levels, and improve the overall health of the heart.

**2. Garlic:** Garlic is another potent herb known for its heart-healthy properties. It contains compounds that can help reduce blood pressure, lower cholesterol levels, and prevent blood clots. Garlic can also improve blood circulation and lower the risk of cardiovascular disease.

**3. Ginger:** Ginger is a popular herb with anti-inflammatory and antioxidant properties, making it excellent for heart health. Ginger can help lower cholesterol levels, reduce blood pressure, and improve blood circulation. Additionally, ginger can help prevent blood clots and improve overall heart health.

**4. Turmeric:** Turmeric is a powerful herb with potent anti-inflammatory properties. It can help prevent plaque buildup in arteries and reduce the risk of heart attack and stroke. Turmeric can also help lower cholesterol levels and improve blood circulation.

**5. Green tea:** Green tea is an antioxidant-rich herb that can help improve heart health. It can reduce the risk of heart disease by improving blood flow and lowering LDL cholesterol levels. Green tea also contains compounds that can help lower blood pressure and prevent blood clots.

In conclusion, herbal remedies can be a potent addition to your heart health routine. However, it is essential to consult with a healthcare professional before adding any new herbals to your diet. Certain herbs can interact with medications or have adverse side effects. Choosing the right herbal remedy can help improve heart health and reduce the risk of cardiovascular disease.

## Nutritional supplements

Nutritional supplements can be a valuable addition to a heart-healthy diet and lifestyle. Here are a few examples of supplements that may support heart health:

**1. Omega-3 fatty acids:** Omega-3s are a type of healthy fat found in oily fish, such as salmon, as well as in some seeds and nuts. They have been shown to support heart health by reducing inflammation, lowering triglycerides, and improving blood pressure.

**2. Coenzyme Q10 (CoQ10):** CoQ10 is an antioxidant that the body naturally produces. It plays a role in energy production in cells and may protect against oxidative damage. Some studies have suggested that CoQ10 supplementation may reduce blood pressure and improve heart function in people with heart failure.

**3. Magnesium:** Magnesium is an important mineral that plays a role in many bodily functions, including muscle and nerve function, as well as heart health. Some studies have linked magnesium supplementation with reduced risk of heart disease, as well as improvements in blood pressure and cholesterol levels.

**4. Vitamin D:** Vitamin D is important for bone health, but it may also play a role in heart health.

Some studies have linked low levels of vitamin D with an increased risk of heart disease, while others have found that vitamin D supplementation may improve blood pressure and cholesterol levels.

It is critical to remember that supplements are not a substitute for a balanced food and lifestyle. If you're considering adding supplements to your routine, be sure to talk to a healthcare professional first to ensure they're right for you.

# CONCLUSION

## Summary of Key Points

**1. Maintaining a healthy diet:** A diet high in fruits, vegetables, whole grains, lean proteins, and healthy fats can help reduce the risk of heart disease.

**2. Regular exercise:** Regular exercise can help lower blood pressure, improve cholesterol levels, and reduce the risk of heart disease.

**3. Cigarette smoking:** Cigarette smoking is a risk factor for heart disease and should be avoided.

**4. Limiting alcohol consumption:** Excessive alcohol consumption can lead to high blood pressure, cardiomyopathy, and other heart conditions.

**5. Stress management:** Chronic stress can increase the risk of heart disease. Managing stress through meditation, yoga, or other relaxation techniques can help lower the risk.

**6. Maintaining a healthy weight:** Being overweight or obese can increase the risk of heart disease. Maintaining a healthy weight through a healthy diet and regular exercise can help lower the risk.

**7. Managing high blood pressure:** High blood pressure is a major risk factor for heart disease. Regular blood pressure checks and medication can help manage hypertension.

**8. Managing cholesterol levels:** High cholesterol levels can increase the risk of heart disease. A healthy diet and medication can help manage cholesterol levels.

**9. Managing diabetes:** Diabetes is a risk factor for heart disease. Managing blood sugar levels through medication and lifestyle changes can help reduce the risk.

**10. Taking medication as prescribed:** If prescribed medication for heart disease or related conditions, it is important to take them as directed by a healthcare professional.

## Future outlook for preventing and reversing heart disease

The future outlook for preventing and reversing heart disease is promising, with advancements in medical research and technology leading to new and innovative approaches. As heart disease continues to be a leading cause of mortality worldwide, efforts to prevent and treat this condition are paramount.

One of the key areas of focus in the future will be personalised medicine. Researchers are working towards developing individualised treatment plans and preventive strategies based on an individual's genetic makeup, lifestyle, and medical history. By identifying specific risk factors and tailoring interventions to suit each person, it is believed that the incidence and progression of heart disease can be significantly reduced.

Advancements in imaging techniques will also play a crucial role in detecting and managing heart disease. Techniques such as coronary artery calcium scoring and cardiac magnetic resonance imaging (MRI) are increasingly being used for early detection and precise assessment of the disease. These non-invasive imaging methods provide valuable information about the extent and severity of arterial blockages, allowing physicians to intervene at an early stage and prevent further damage.

Furthermore, the field of regenerative medicine offers promising potential in the future. Researchers are exploring ways to regenerate damaged heart tissue using stem cells, tissue engineering, and other advanced techniques. This could provide a revolutionary solution for reversing the effects of heart disease and restoring normal heart function.

In addition, advancements in digital health technologies and telemedicine will enable better monitoring and management of heart disease. Wearable devices, smartphone applications, and remote patient monitoring systems allow for real-time tracking of vital signs and early detection of any abnormalities. Telemedicine platforms enable patients to consult with healthcare professionals remotely, ensuring regular follow-ups and timely intervention.

The future outlook also includes a strong emphasis on lifestyle modifications and preventive measures. Continued efforts to educate individuals about the importance of a healthy diet, regular exercise, stress management, and smoking cessation will contribute to reducing the incidence of heart disease. Additionally, campaigns aimed at promoting awareness and early detection through regular screenings will play a vital role in preventing the development of advanced stages of heart disease.

In conclusion, the future outlook for preventing and reversing heart disease is promising. By integrating personalised medicine, advanced imaging techniques, regenerative medicine, digital health technologies, and lifestyle modifications, there is hope for a significant reduction in the burden of heart disease. Continued research and developments in these areas will ultimately lead to improved outcomes, enhanced quality of life, and a healthier population.

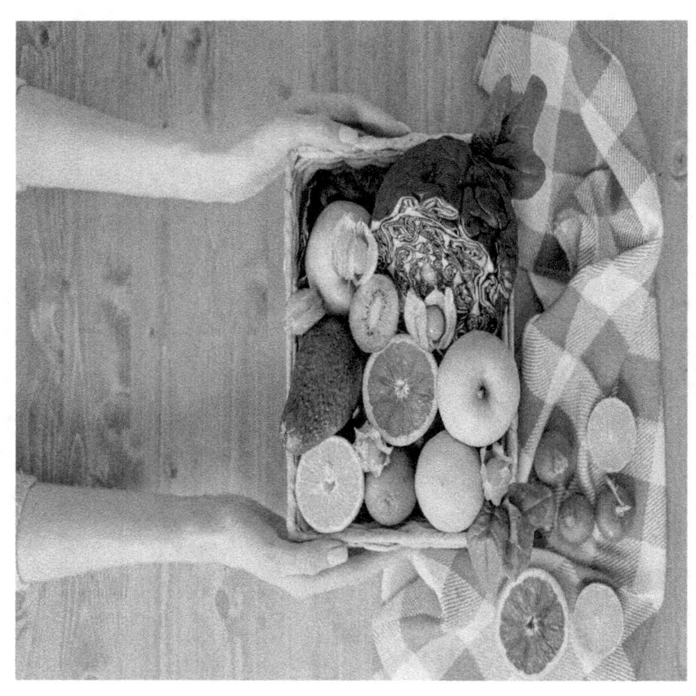